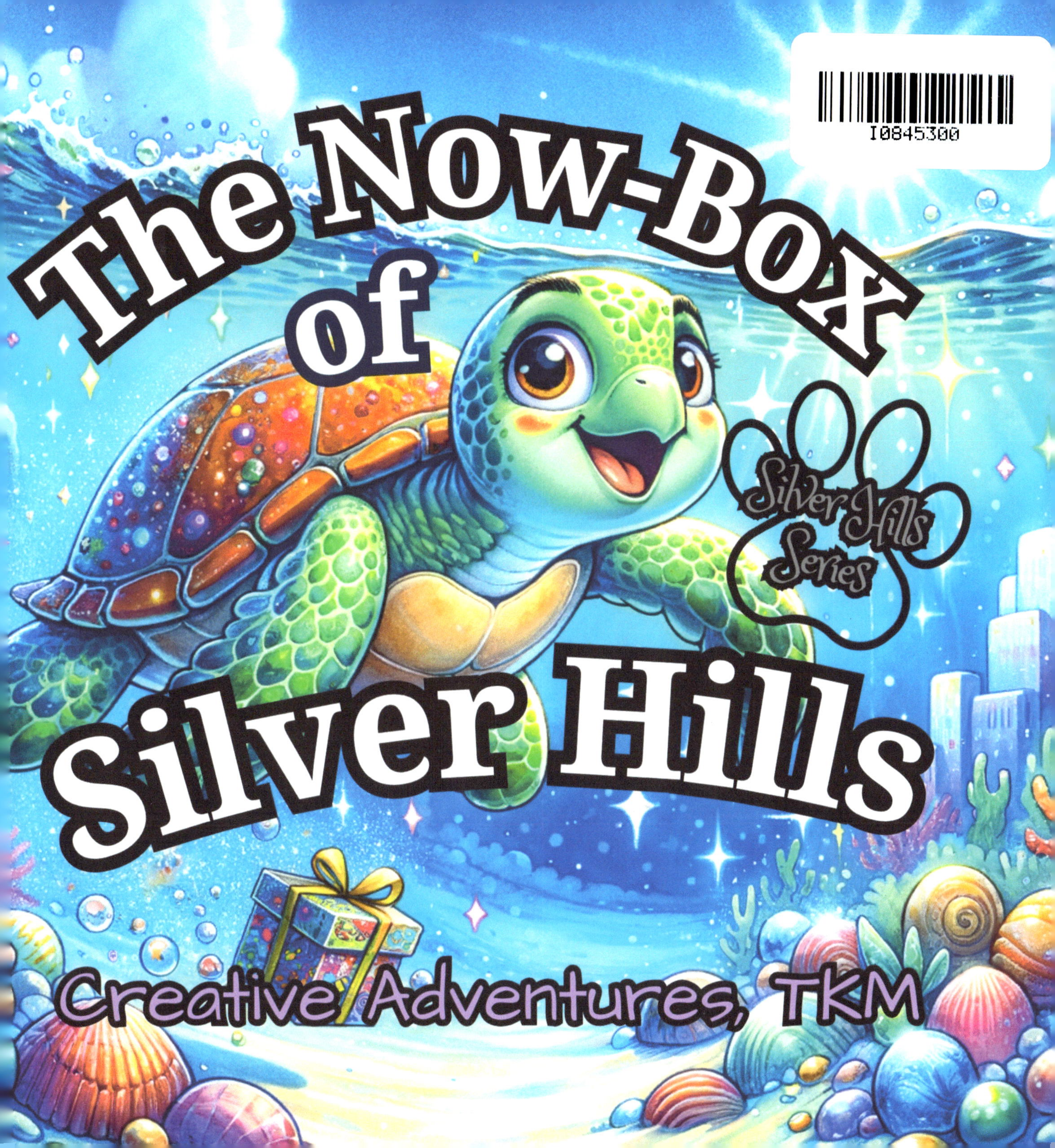

The Now-Box of
Silver Hills
Silver Hills Series
Creative Adventures, TKM
I0845300

Copyright © 2024 by Tanya Moore / Creative Adventures, TKM. All rights reserved.

This book or any portion thereof may not be reproduced or used in any manner whatsoever without the express written permission of the author or publisher except for the use of brief quotations in a book review.

Disclaimer and Terms of Use:

The Author and Publisher has strived to be as accurate and complete as possible in the creation of this book, notwithstanding the fact that she does not warrant or represent at any time that the contents within are accurate due to the rapidly changing nature of the Internet. While all attempts have been made to verify information provided in this publication, the Author and Publisher assume no responsibility for errors, omissions, or contrary interpretation of the subject matter herein. Any perceived slights of specific persons, peoples, or organizations are unintentional.

This book or any portion thereof may not be reproduced or used in any manner whatsoever without the express written permission of the author or publisher except for the use of brief quotations in a book review.

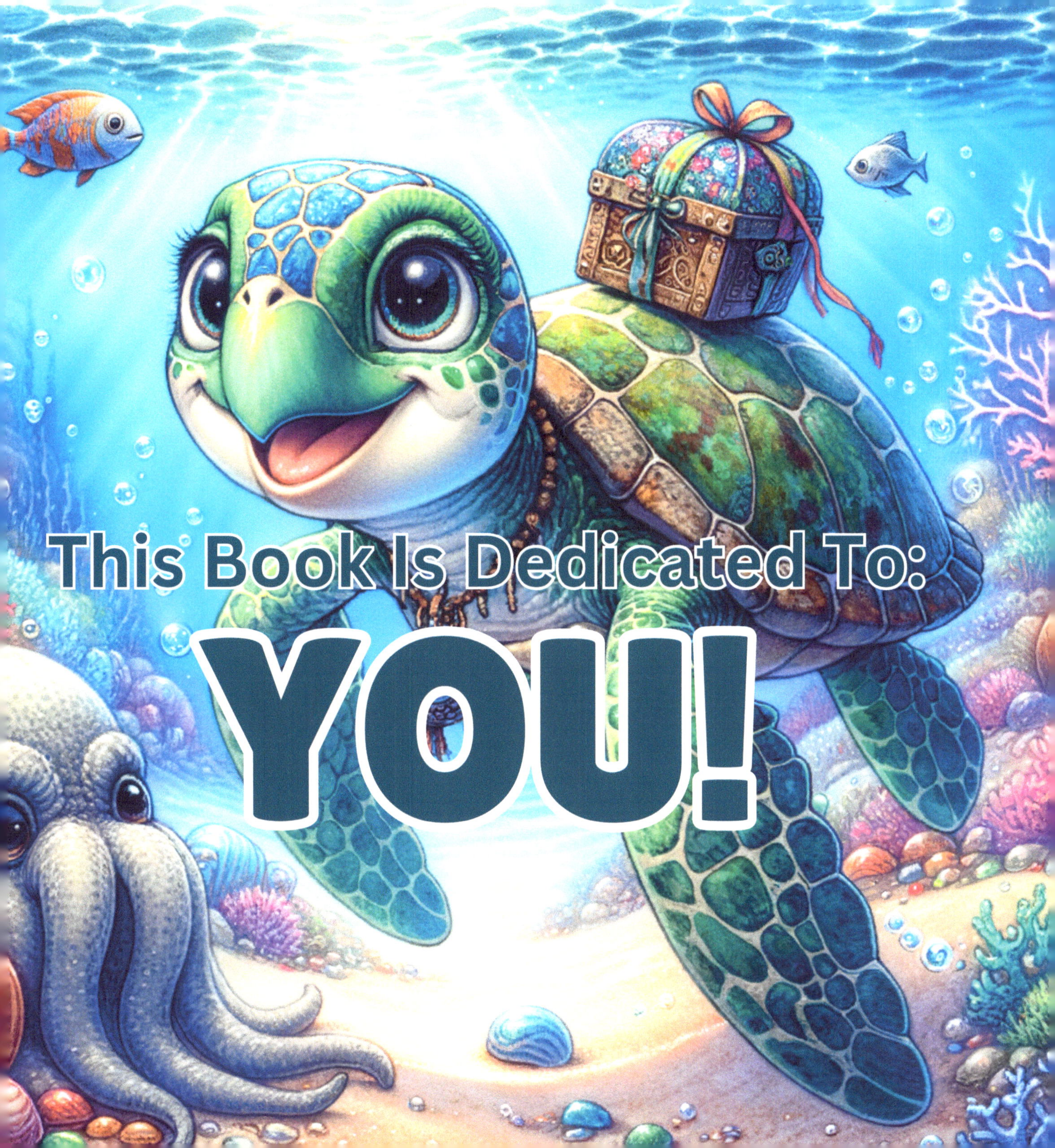

This Book Is Dedicated To:
YOU!

Fanta the Sea-turtle swam through the sparkling ocean, her shiny green shell gleaming in the sunlight.

On top of her hard shell, she carried a curious box labeled 'Now'.

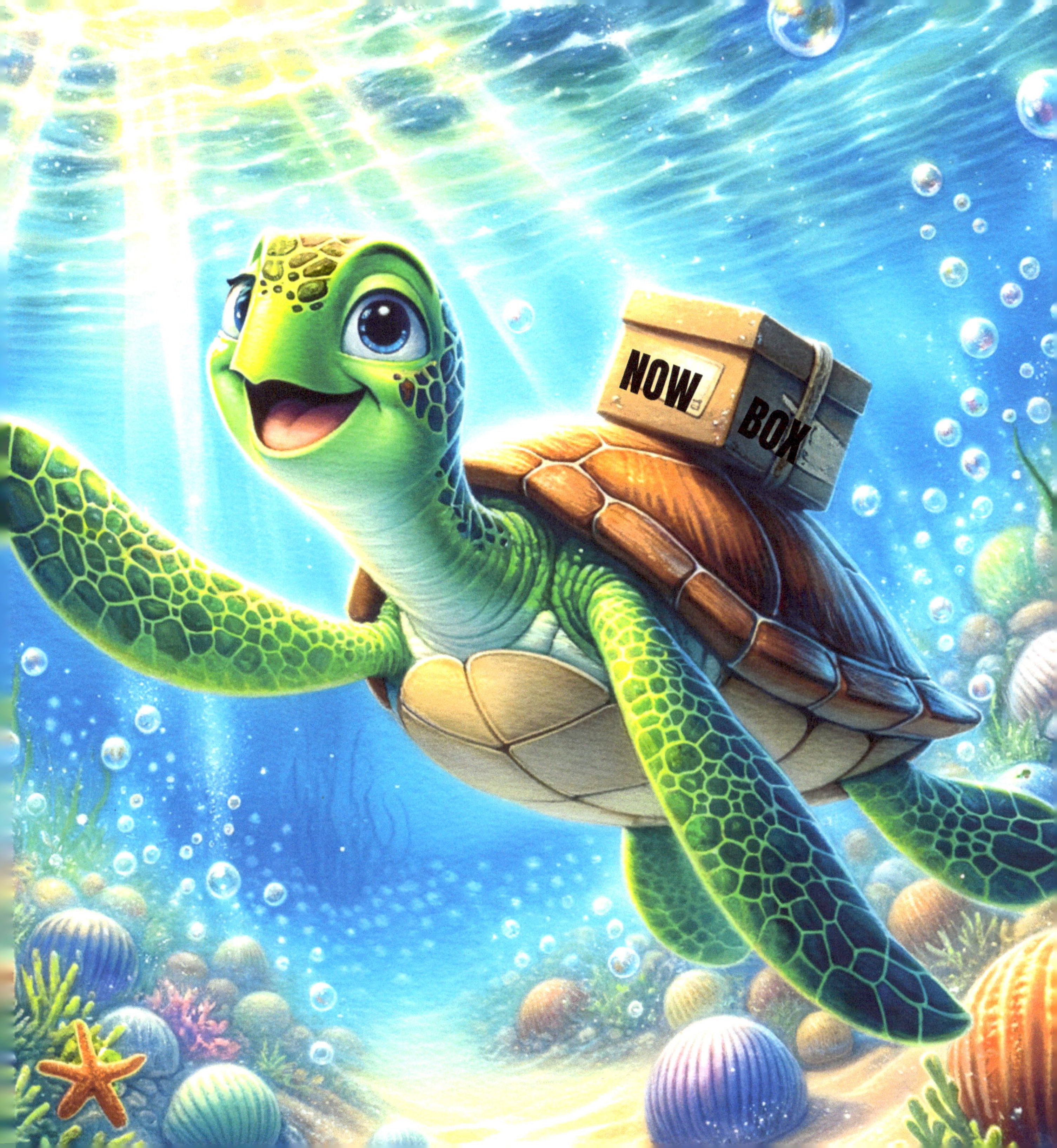

NOW
BOX

As she approached the sandy beaches of Silver Hills, a quaint community for elderly sea creatures, Fanta pondered, "I wonder what this Now-Box is for?"

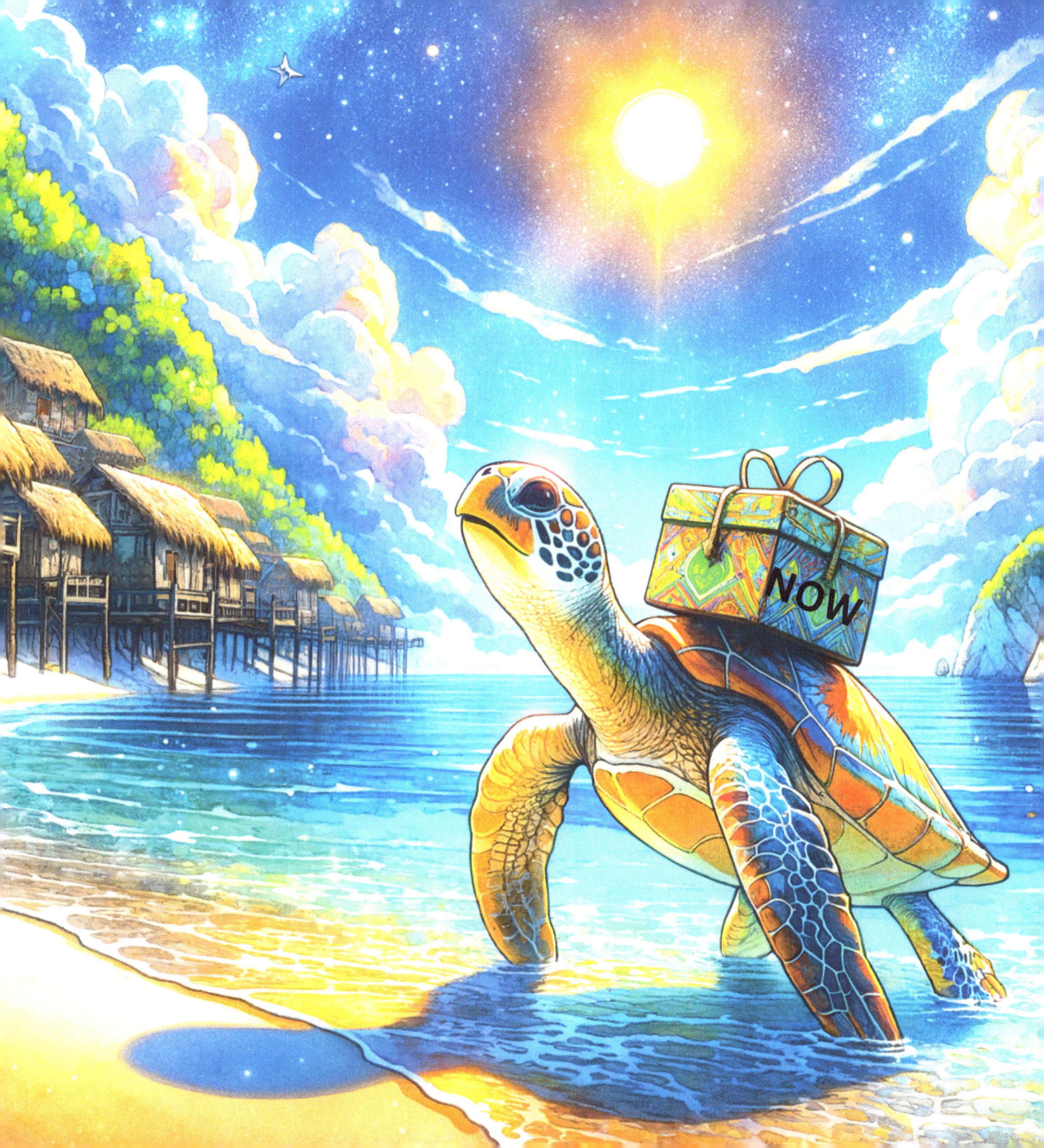

NOW

Upon reaching the shore, Fanta was greeted by a colorful array of old friends—elderly fish, octopuses, and even a couple of hefty, yet gentle whales.

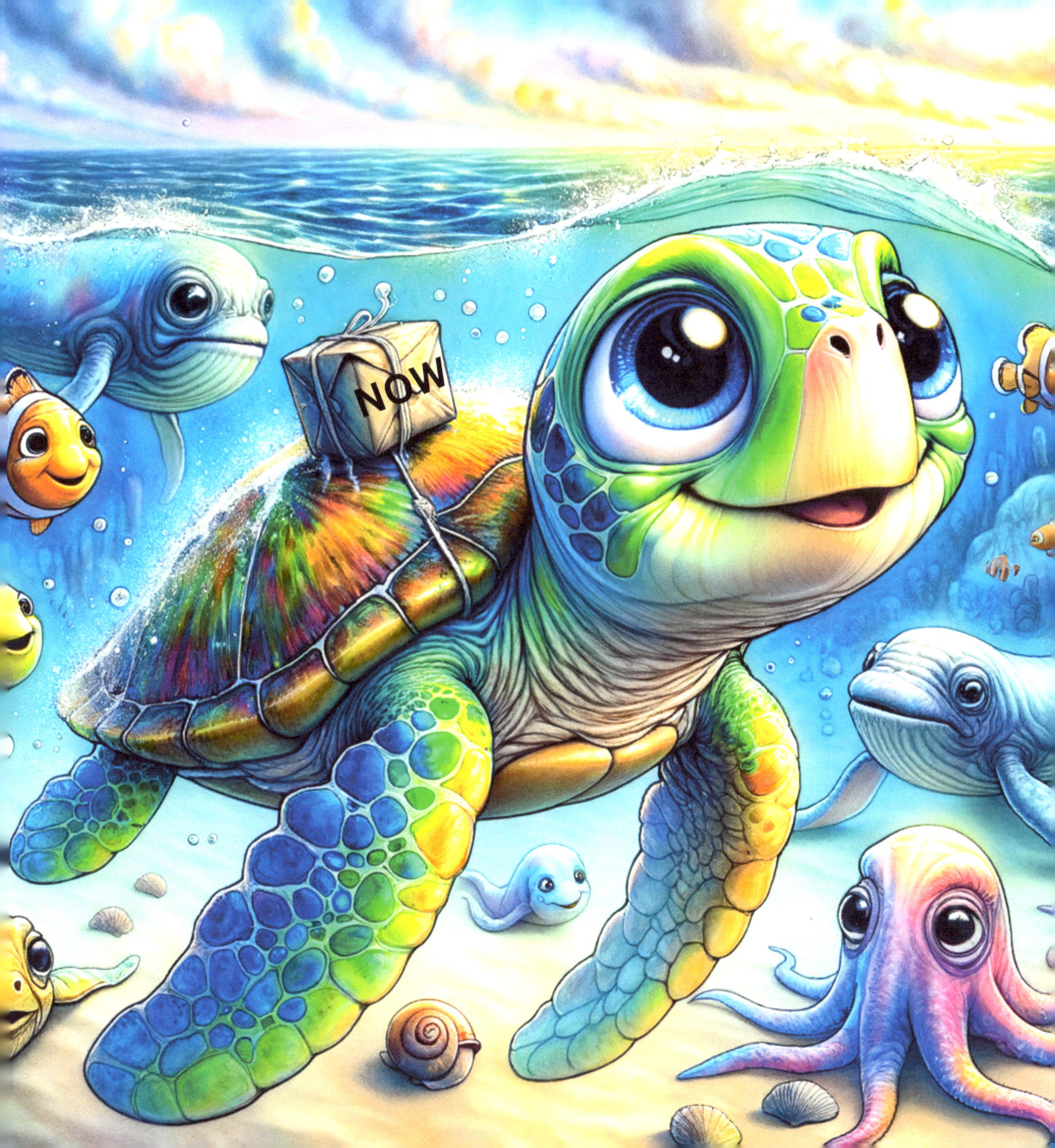
NOW

With a wide smile, Fanta announced, "Hello, everyone! I've brought a special surprise — a Now Box!"

Curious eyes and tentacles gathered around, eager to discover its secrets.

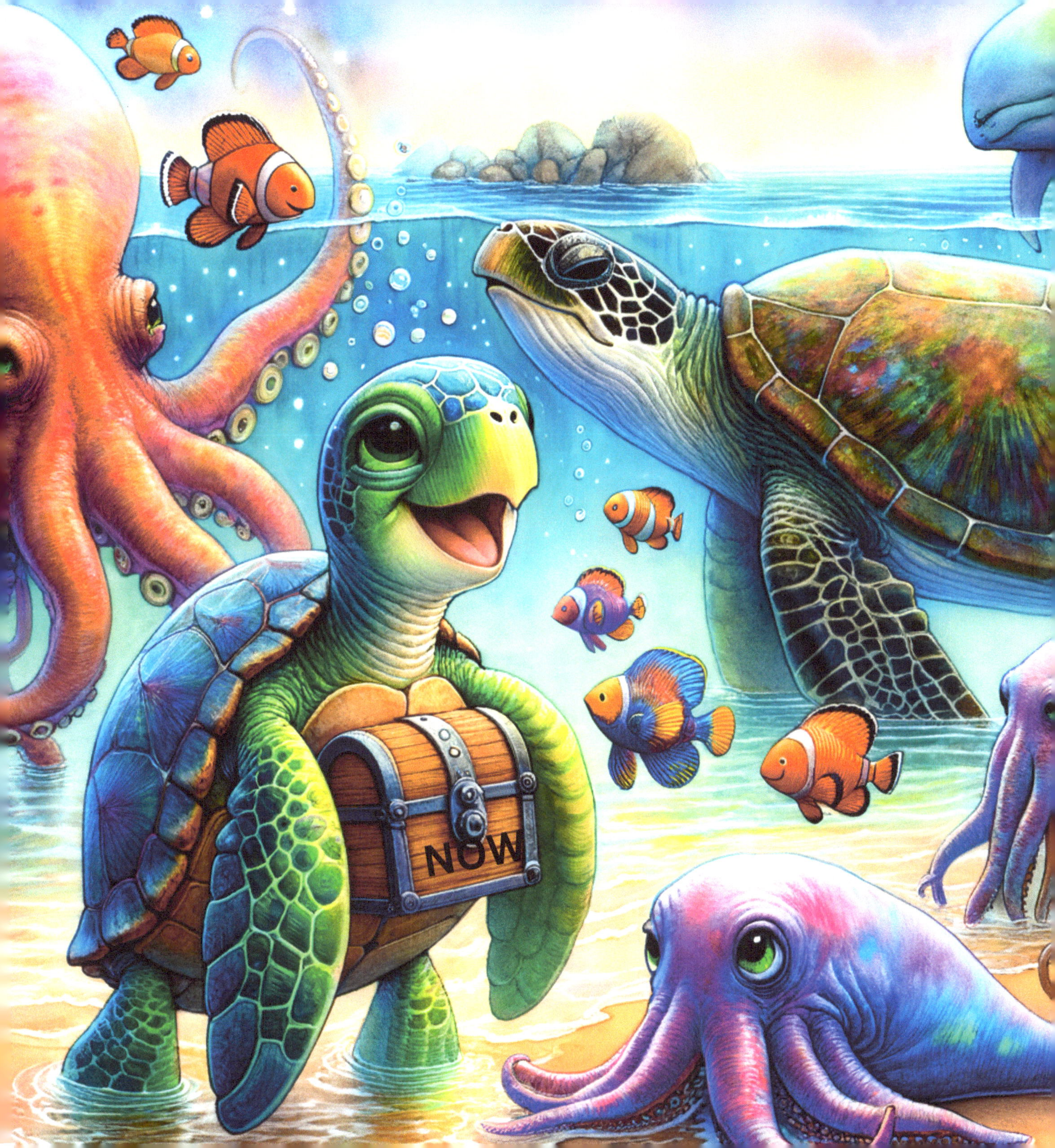
NOW

Mrs. Octopus, always full of ideas, suggested, "Let's fill it with our cherished memories!"

She tried dropping a shiny pearl into the box, but it slipped right through!

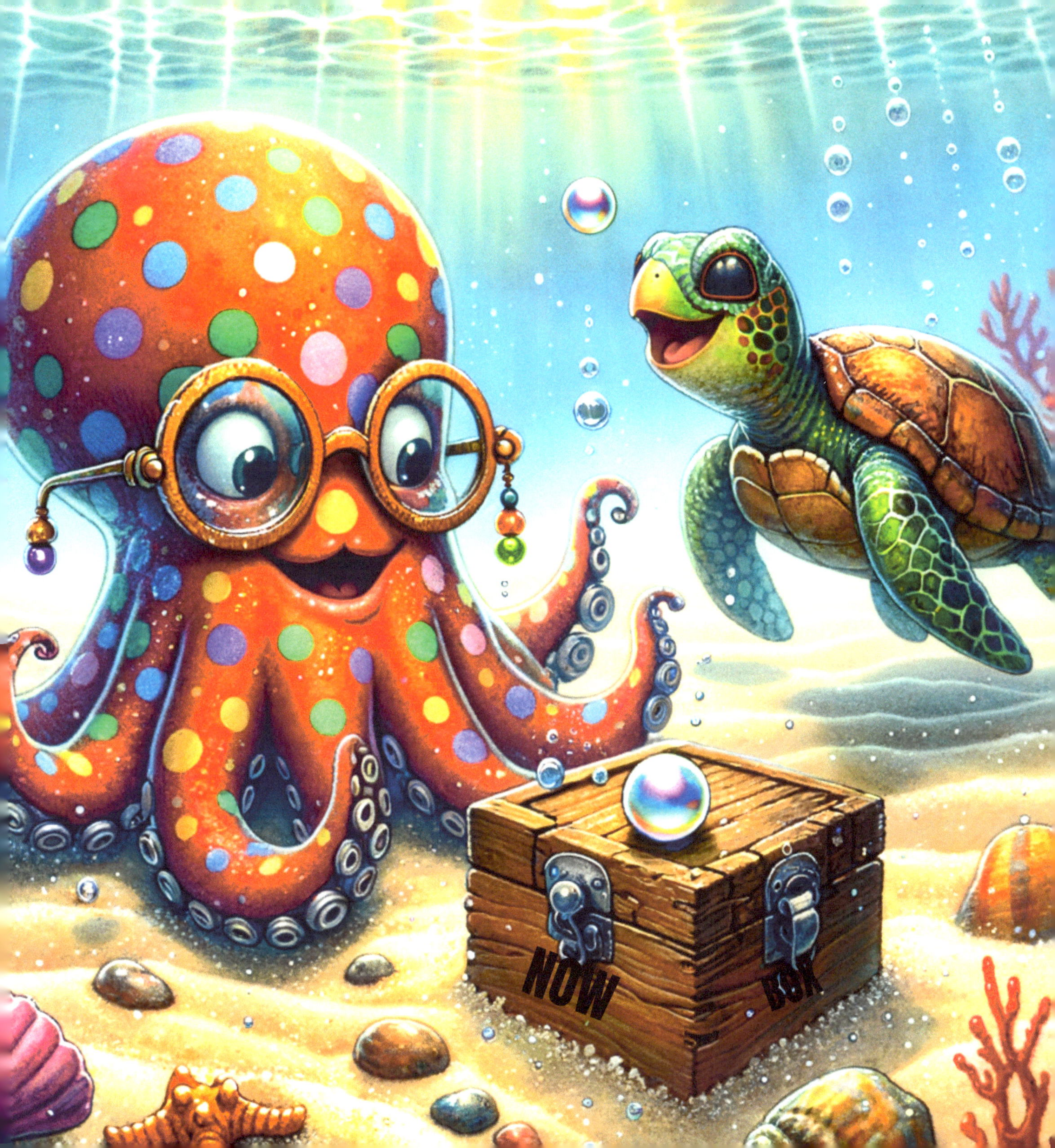

NOW
BOK

Laughing heartily, Mr. Whale proposed, "Perhaps it's designed for our future dreams!"

He whispered a dream of a vast ocean journey into the box, but his words, like mist, vanished into the air.

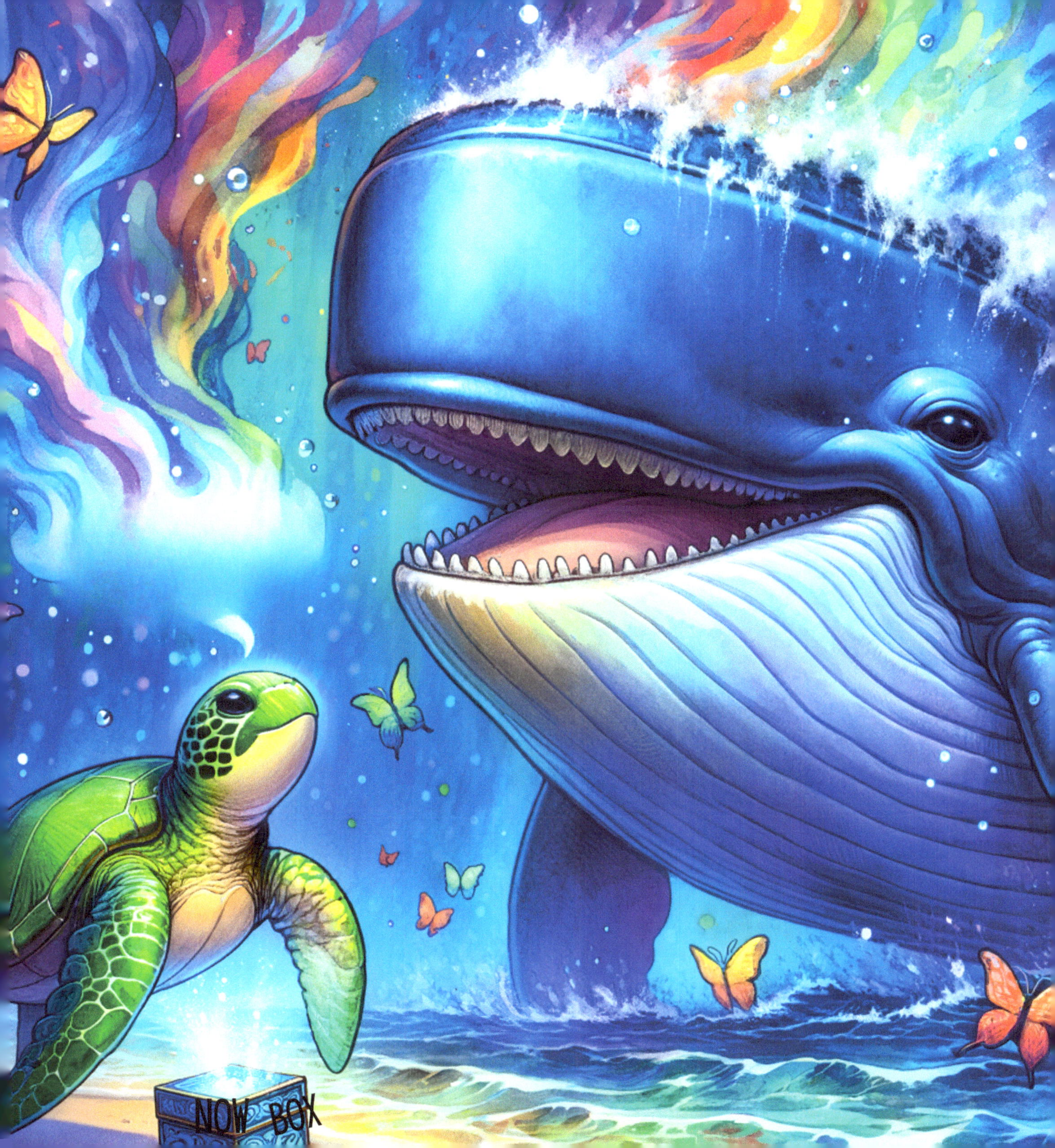
NOW BOX

A murmur of confusion rippled through the group.

"What could this peculiar Now-Box be for?" they whispered amongst themselves.

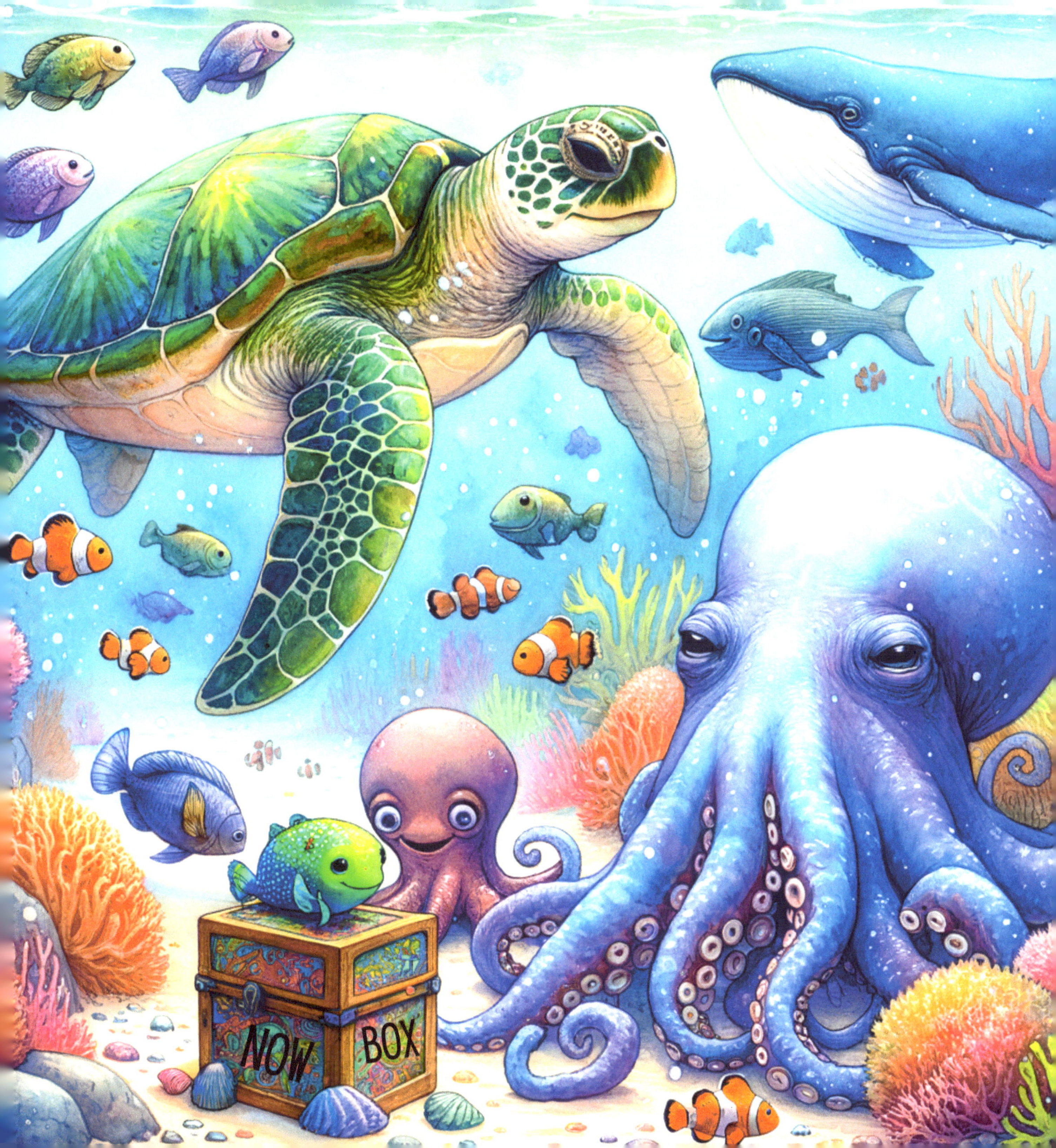
NOW   BOX

Just then, a wise old crab scuttled over. His eyes twinkled as he looked at the Now-Box.

"My friends," he said softly, "this box isn't for the past or the future. It's for right now!"

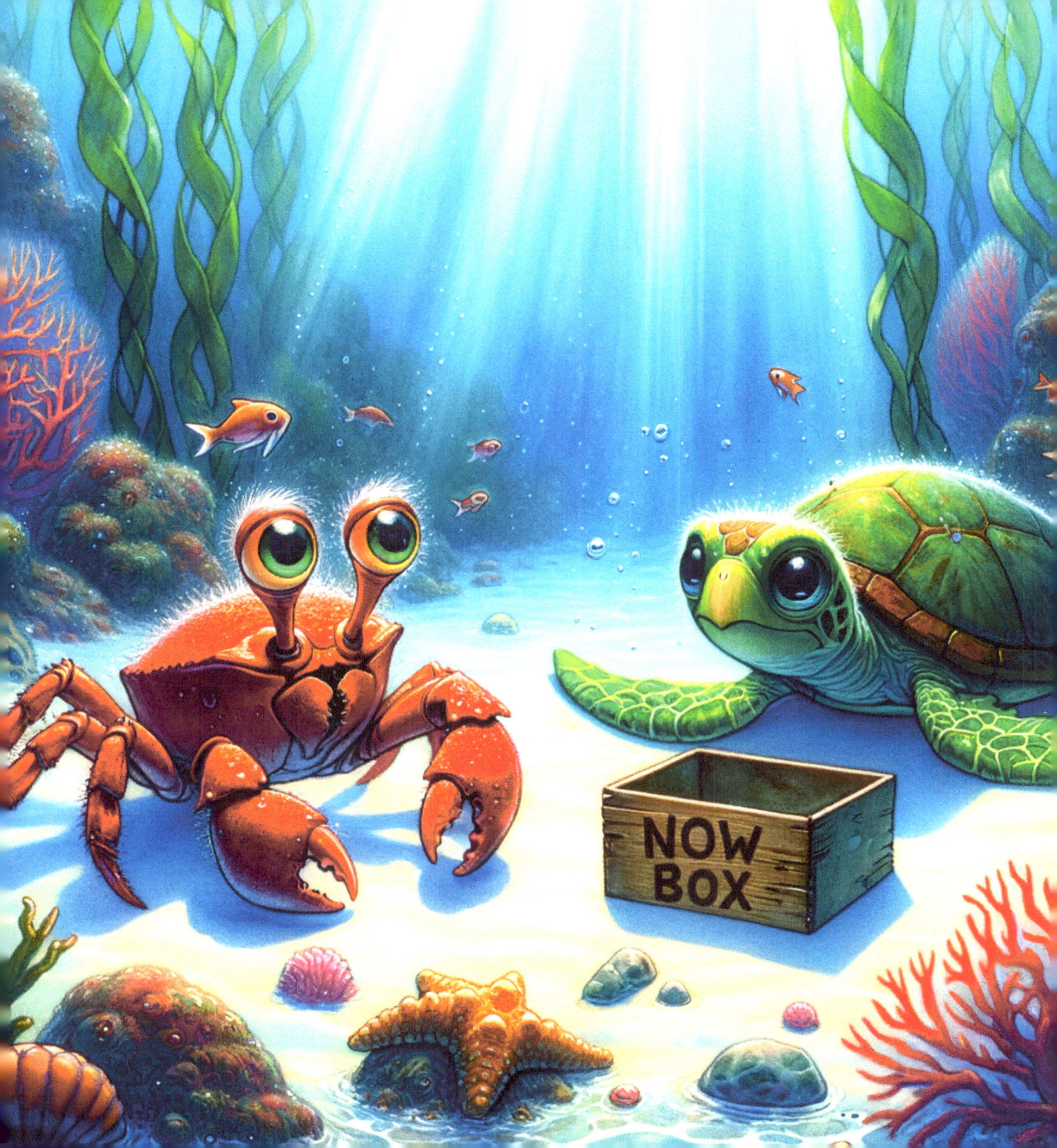

NOW
BOX

The crab gently took the box and held
it up to the warm sun.

"Look closely," he said. "What do you
see?"

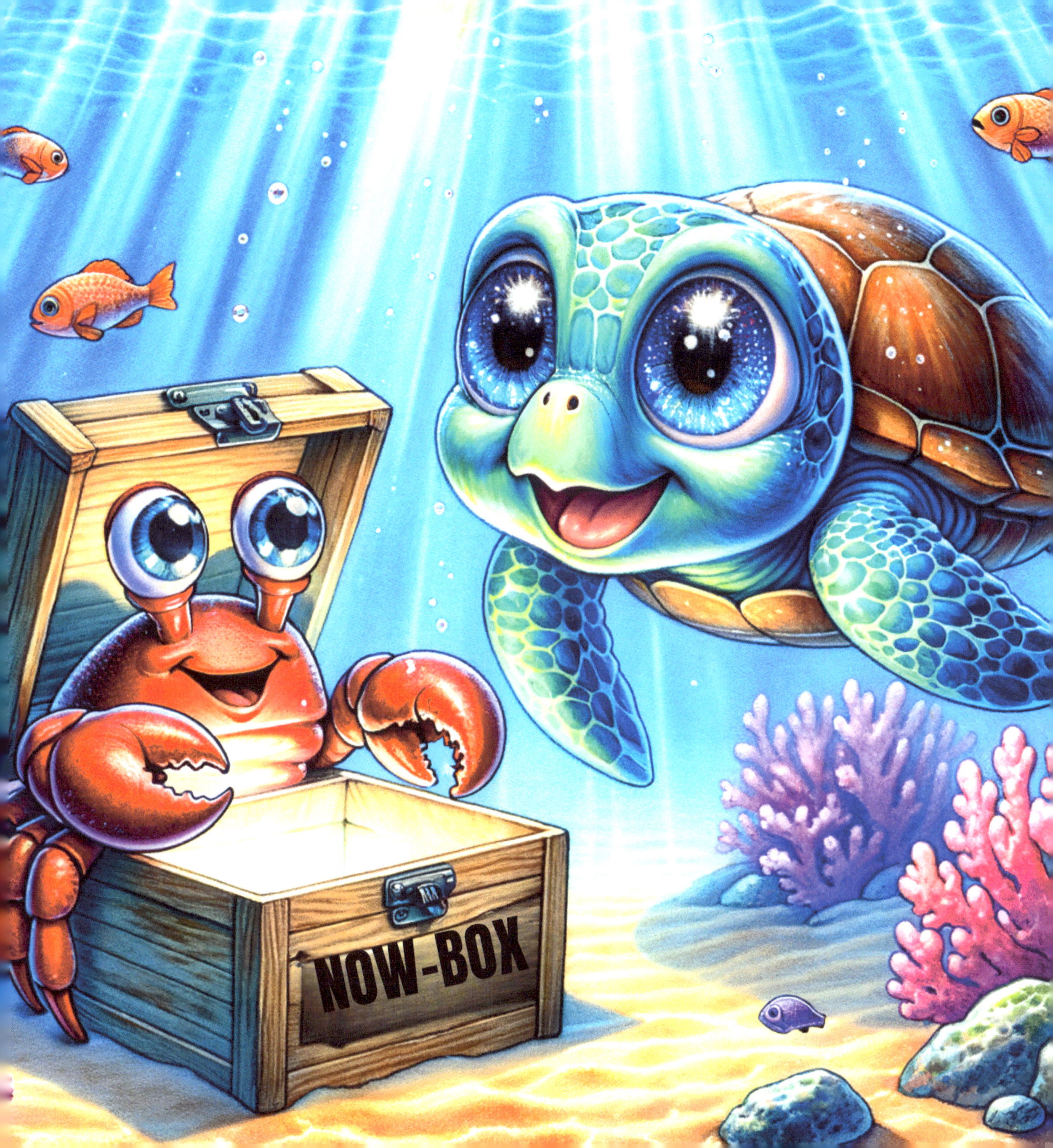
NOW-BOX

To everyone's amazement, a soft golden light began to glow inside the box.

"That's the light of the present moment," the crab explained. "It's always there, waiting for us to notice it."

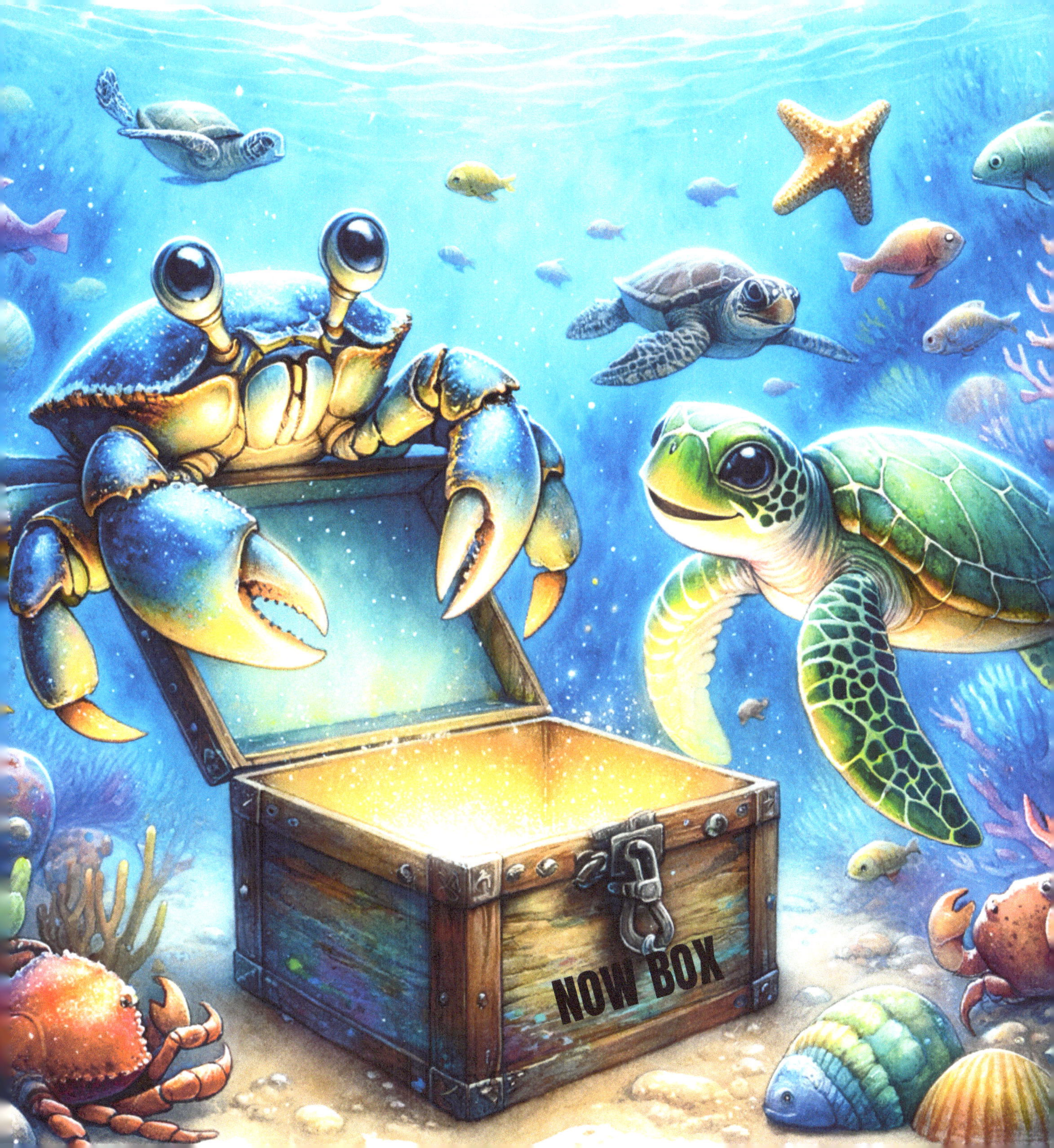
NOW BOX

Inspired, Mrs. Octopus felt the warm rays on her skin.

"It's in the simple joy of feeling the sun," she realized.

Mr. Whale agreed, adding, "And in hearing the soothing whisper of the waves."

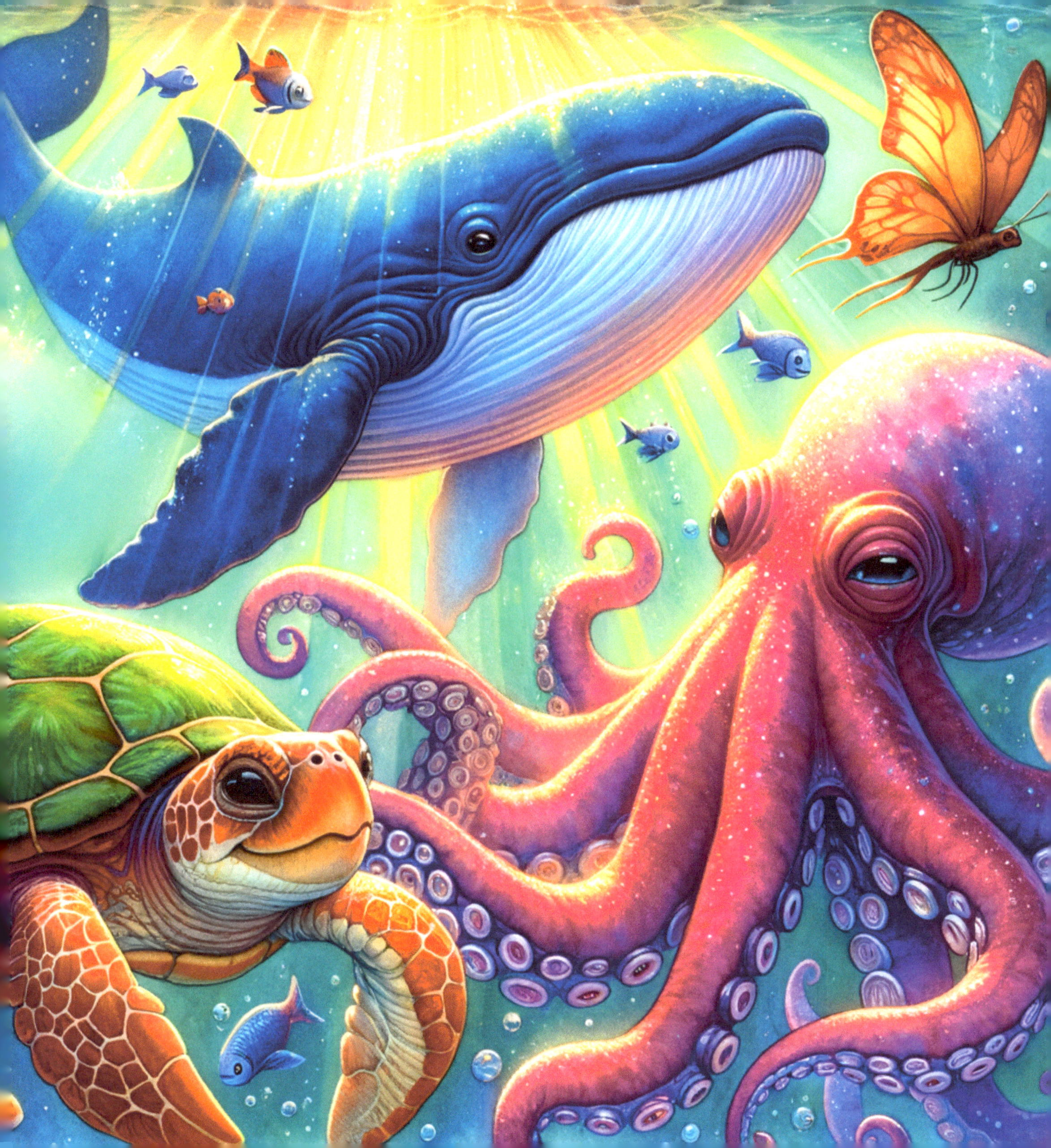

Soon, all the residents of Silver Hills were pointing out golden moments:

The taste of salty sea air, the laughter of friends, the joy of wiggling their fins.

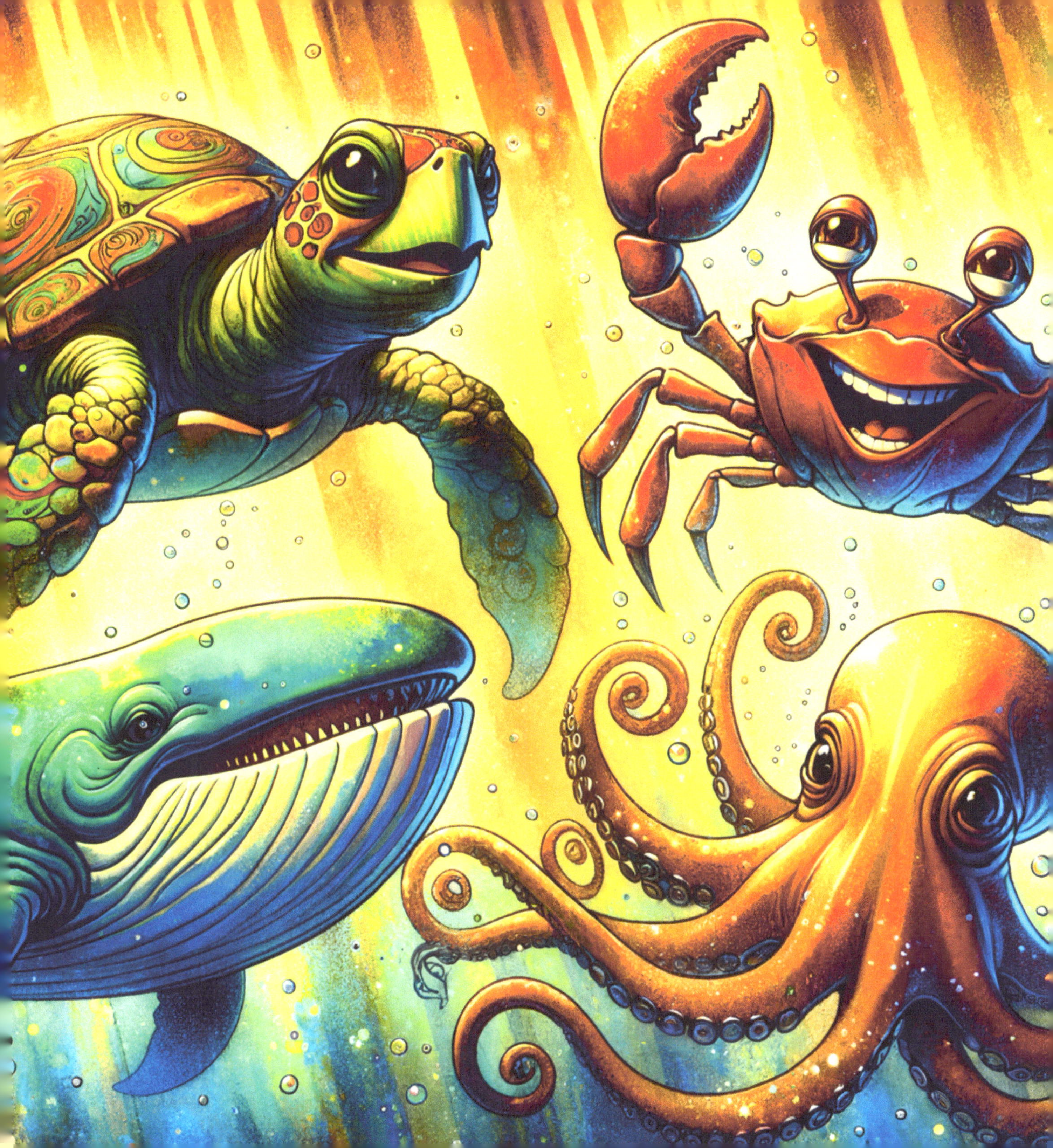

Fanta, heart swelling with joy, proclaimed, "Our Now Box is indeed full, overflowing with the magic found right here in the moments we share!"

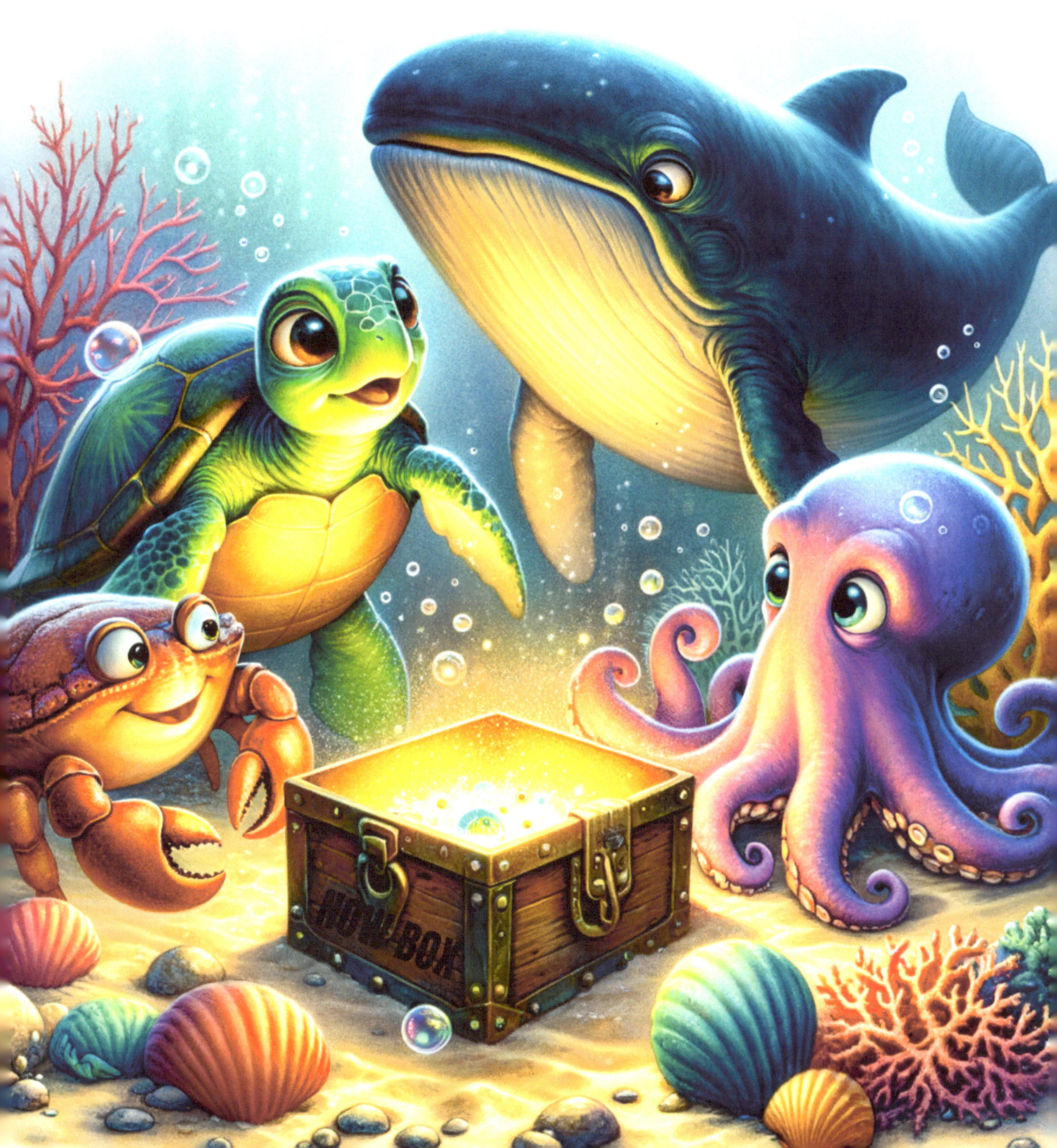

From that day on, the residents of Silver Hills started each morning by sharing their 'golden moments' with each other.

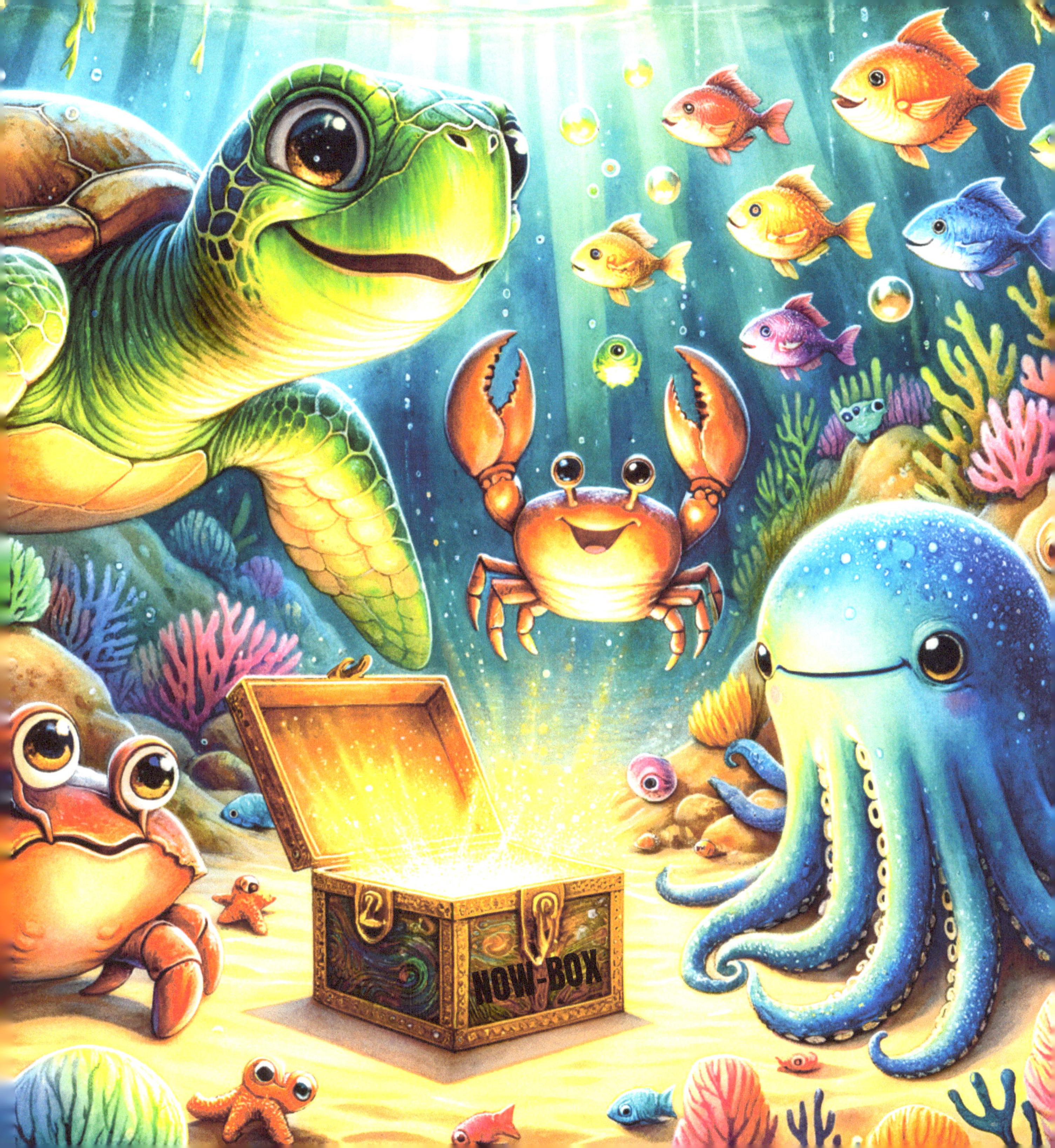
NOW-BOX

A new tradition was born in Silver Hills. Every day, each resident would share a golden moment from their day, which they savored and celebrated in the 'now' moments together.

They discovered that no matter their age, there was always something fun and wonderful happening in the present moment.

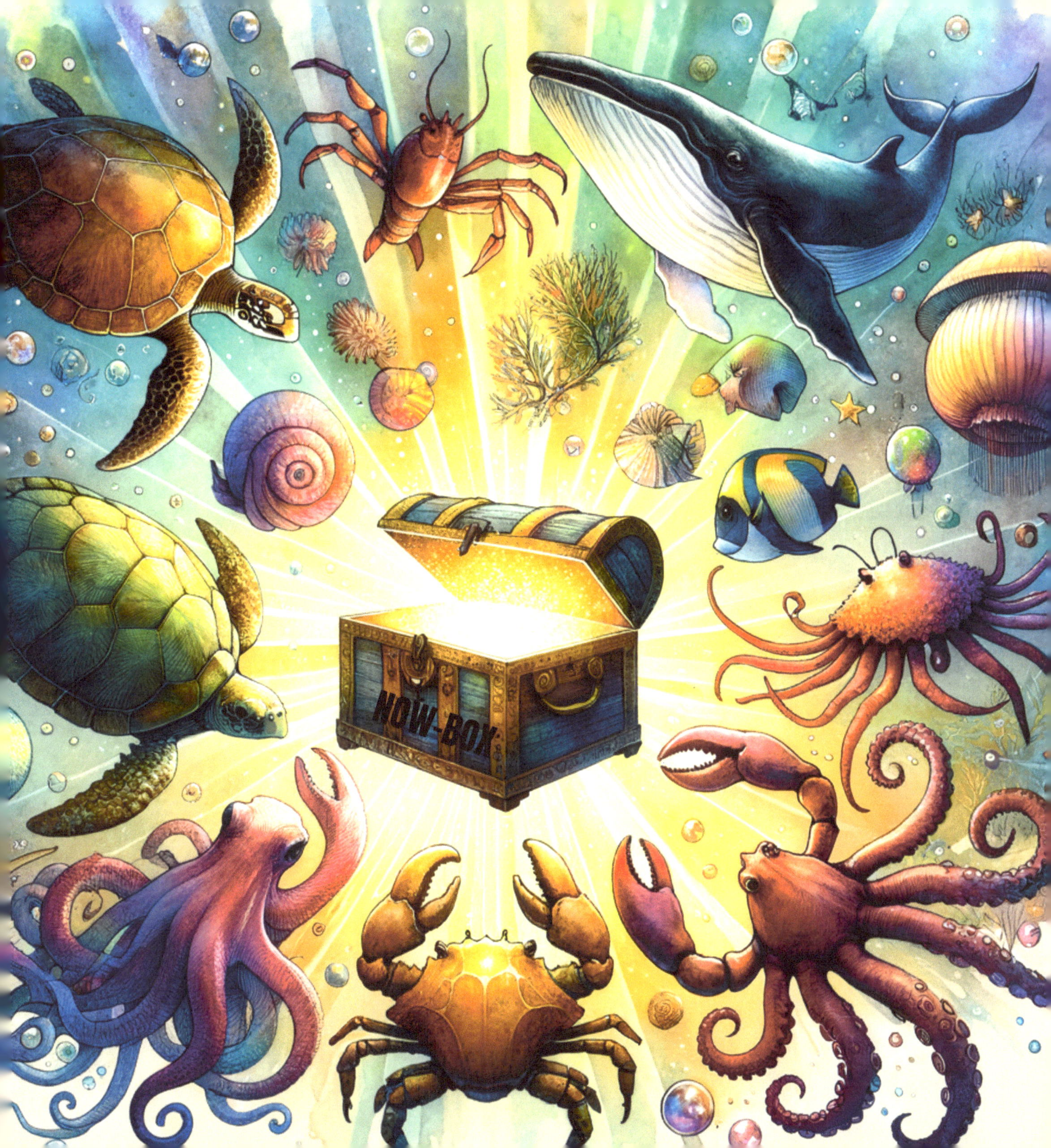
NOW-BOX

As orange and pink hues painted the sky at dusk, Fanta watched her friends bask in laughter and contentment.

The Now-Box had shown them all a treasure beyond price—the joy of living fully in the now.

A treasure more precious than any memory or dream. And so, life at Silver Hills carried on, rich with moments of the Golden Light.

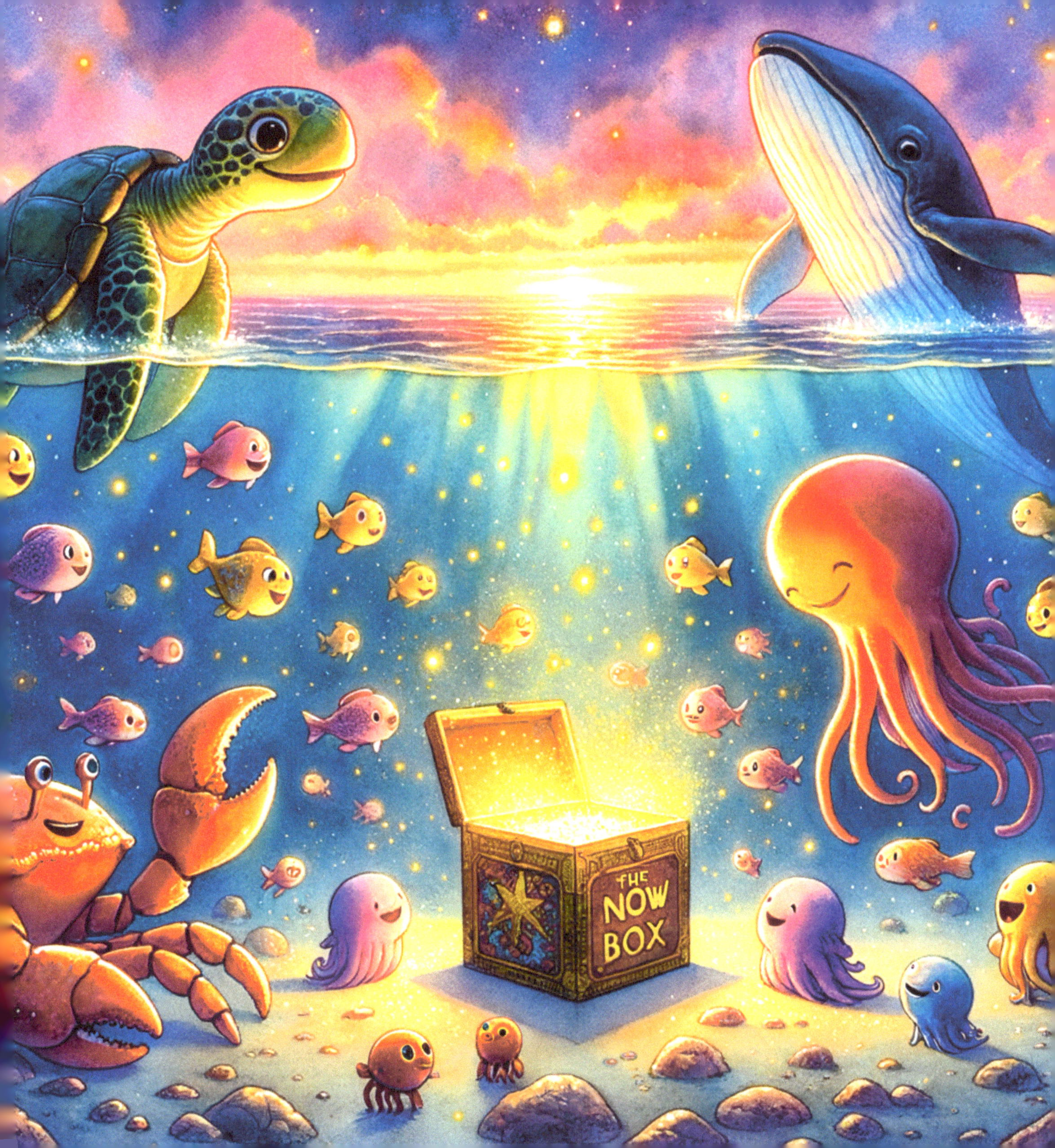

THE
NOW
BOX

FOR YOUR FREE COLORING BOOK PRINTABLE, SCAN QR CODE HERE:
FOR MORE BOOKS FROM THIS AUTHOR, SCAN QR CODE HERE:
Amazon.com/Author/CreativeAdventuresTKM
Amazon.com/Author/TanyaMoore

www.ingramcontent.com/pod-product-compliance
Lightning Source LLC
Chambersburg PA
CBHW040202240726
48664CB00002B/796